Recipes of How Babies are Made

Written by
Carmen Martínez Jover

Illustrations by
Rosemary Martínez

Special thanks
to Diana Guerra, who suggested the
theme of this story. I shall always be grateful
for her support and friendship and to
our daughters Anna and Nicole
who put us on this same path.

Carmen Martinez Jover

To the stars of my life.

Rosemary Martinez

Babies and cakes are made in very similar ways

Ingredients for making a cake:

✓ milk
✓ flour
✓ eggs
✓ butter

+

an oven **=** a cake

Ingredients for making a baby:

a sperm ✓

an egg ✓

a tummy

+

=

a baby

Where do the ingredients for making a cake come from?

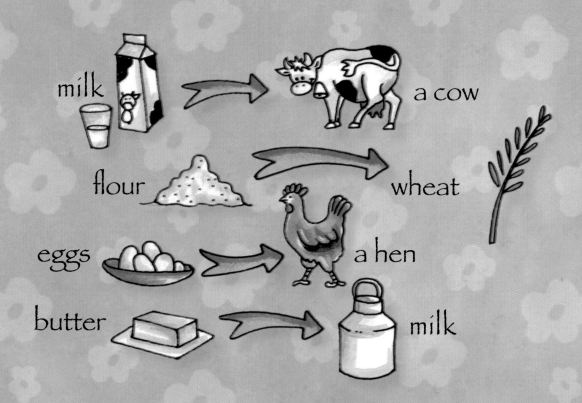

milk → a cow

flour → wheat

eggs → a hen

butter → milk

Instructions:

Mix all the ingredients and place in an oven.

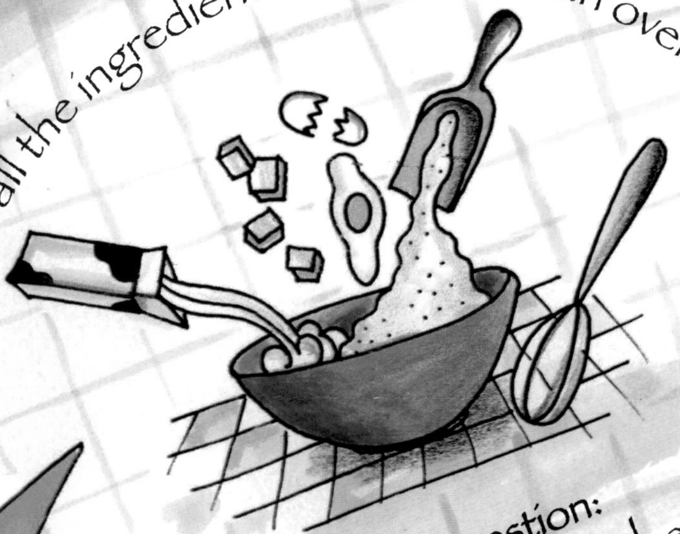

Question:

Where does the cake grow?

Answer:

In an oven and it takes about 30 minutes.

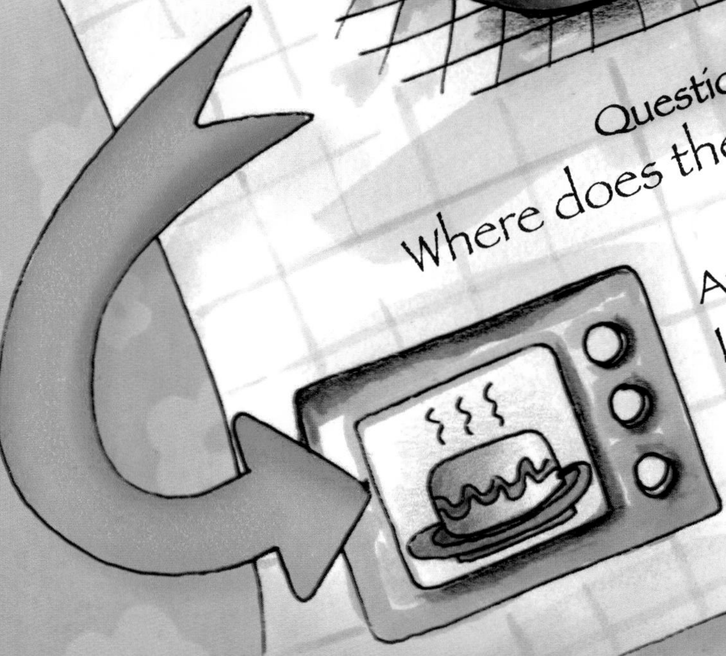

Where do the ingredients for making a baby come from?

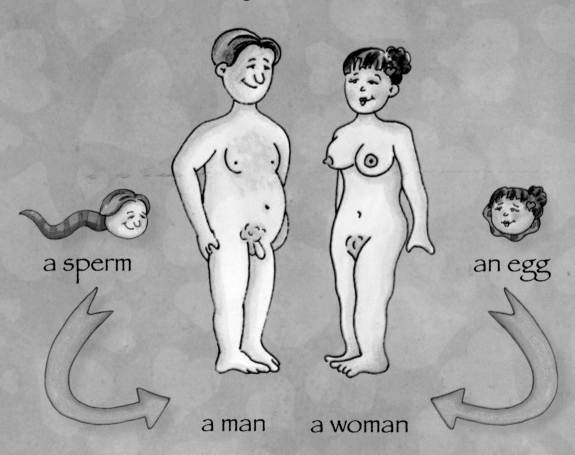

a sperm

a man

a woman

an egg

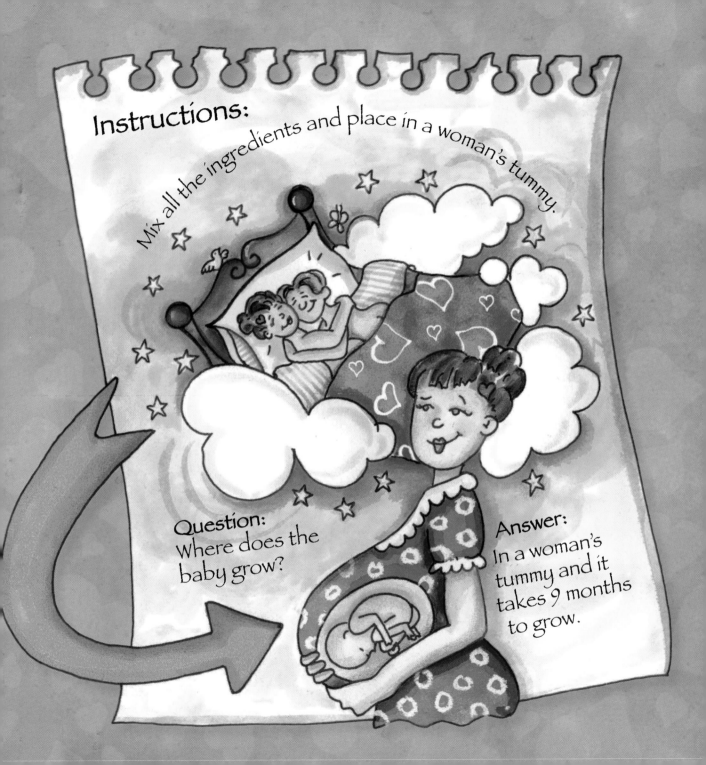

How a baby is formed

Inside a woman's tummy, which we call a **womb**, an **egg** and a **sperm** merge to become **one cell**, when this happens we say they are **fertilized**.

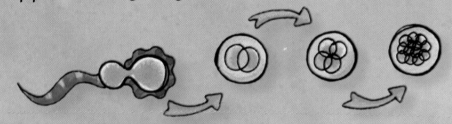

Then the cell starts to grow and divide to form the beginning of a baby, which we call an **embryo**, when it grows bigger we call it a **fetus** and when it is born we call it a **baby**.

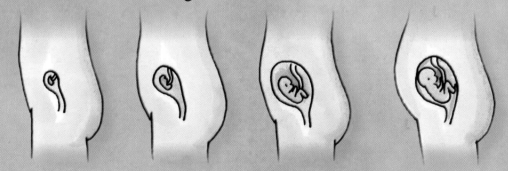

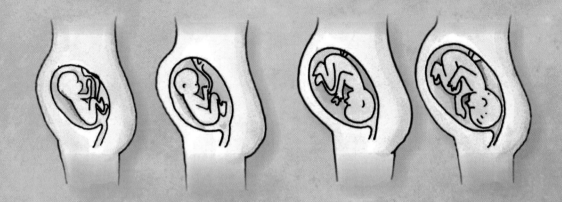

A woman is **pregnant** from the moment of fertilization to the moment of birth. During this time the fetus grows and grows in the womb for **9 months**.

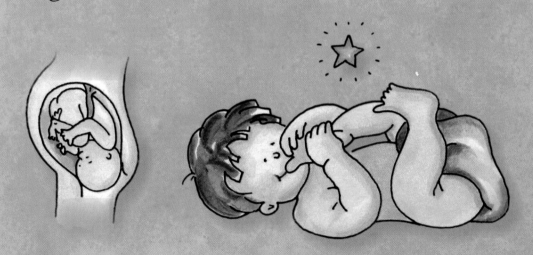

When an ingredient is missing

Sometimes couples want to have
a baby but the "classical recipe" doesn't
seem to work, so they feel very sad
because they really want to have a baby
to become a Mummy and a Daddy.

We are going to tell you about all
the different recipes of how
babies are made.

Let's review what we need for
each recipe:

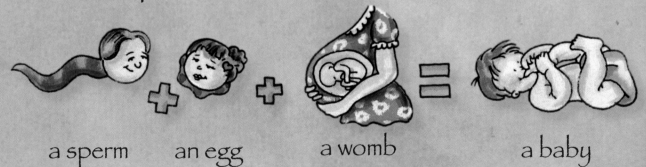

a sperm   an egg   a womb   a baby

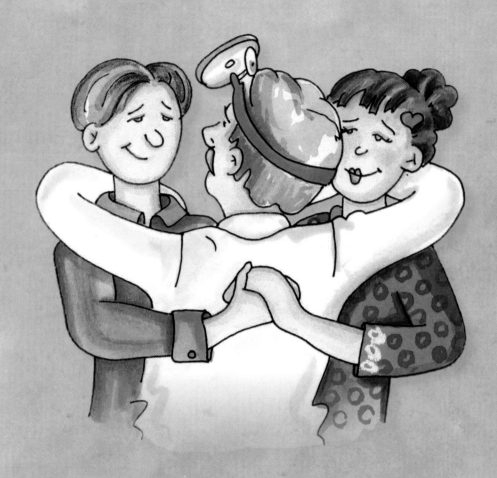

Sometimes Mummy and Daddy do not have these basic ingredients so they look for a doctor to help them have their baby.

Classical recipe

In this recipe, which is also known as **"natural conception"**, Daddy's sperm and Mummy's egg fertilize naturally in Mummy's womb.

"Natural or naturally" means that this happens without the help of a doctor.

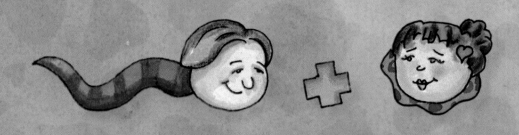

a sperm + an egg

Once the egg is fertilized by the sperm they start dividing, forming an embryo, then it becomes a fetus and then it continues to grow and grow until 9 months later their baby is born.

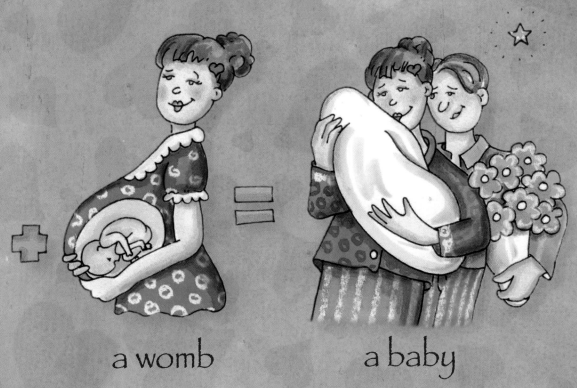

a womb   a baby

In Vitro recipe

Sometimes Mummy's egg and Daddy's sperm don't seem to fertilize by themselves so the doctor puts them together in a test tube and looks after them until they manage to fertilize and become an embryo.

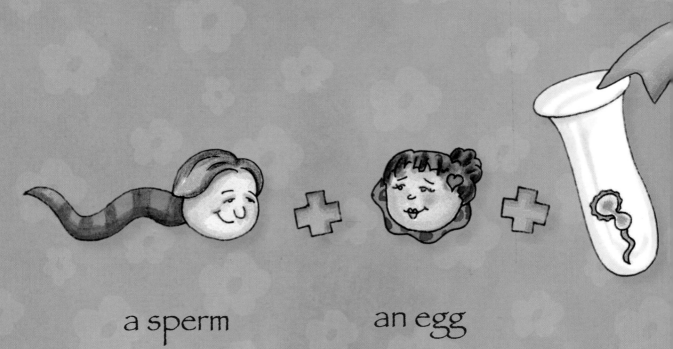

a sperm   an egg

When the embryo starts to grow the doctor puts it into Mummy's womb, where it continues to grow until 9 months later their baby is born.

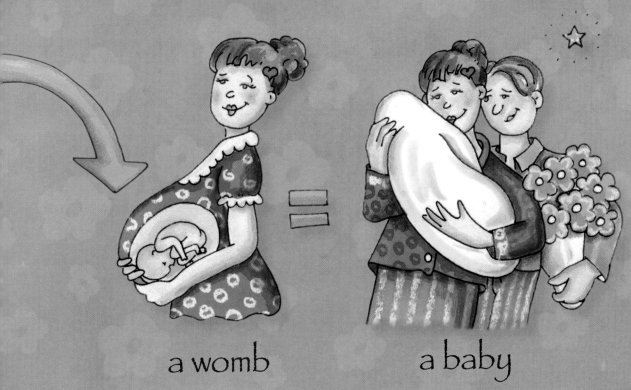

a womb   a baby

Sperm donation recipe

Sometimes Daddy's sperms don't work properly so another man gives him some of his sperms, we call this "sperm donation".

The doctor fertilizes Mummy's egg in a test tube with the donated sperms.

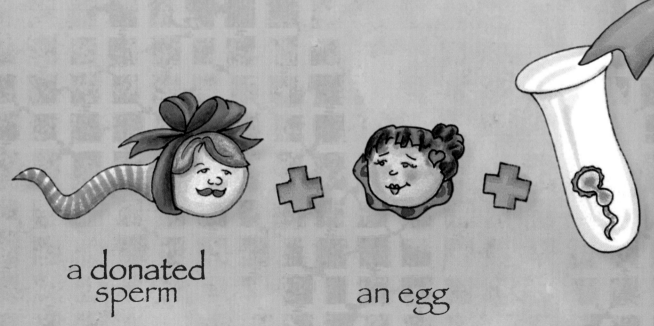

a donated sperm

an egg

When the embryo starts growing the doctor places it in Mummy's womb so it can continue to grow for 9 months until their baby is born.

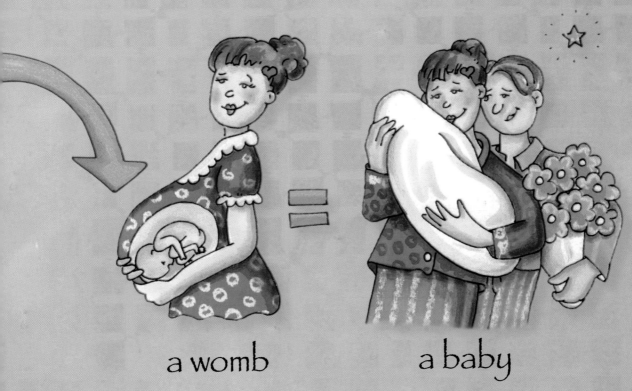

a womb   a baby

Egg donation recipe

Sometimes Mummy's eggs don't work properly so another woman gives her one of her eggs, we call this "egg donation".

The doctor fertilizes the donated egg with Daddy's sperms in a test tube.

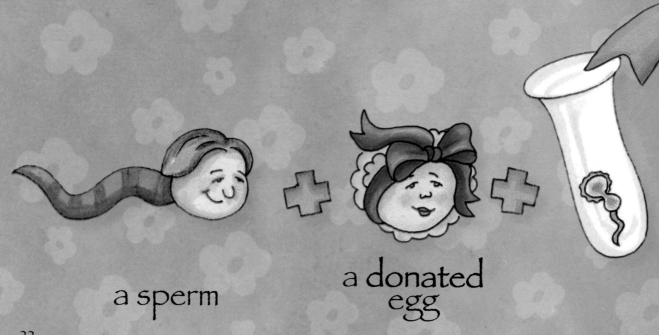

a sperm   a donated egg

When the egg and the sperm fertilize and the embryo starts to grow, the doctor places it in Mummy's womb so that it can continue to grow for 9 months until their baby is born.

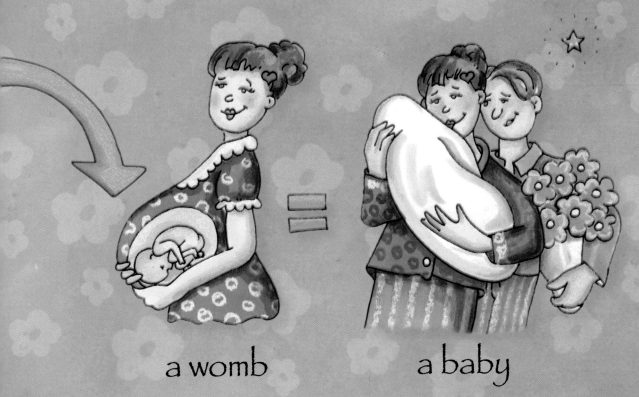

a womb   a baby

Embryo donation

In this recipe Mummy's eggs don't work properly and neither do Daddy's sperms, so another woman donates one of her eggs and another man donates one of his sperms.

The doctor helps the donated eggs and the donated sperms to fertilize in a test tube.

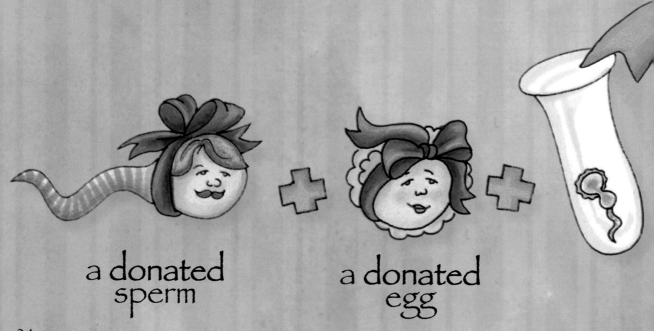

a donated
sperm

a donated
egg

When the embryo starts growing, the doctor places this donated embryo in Mummy's womb, so it can grow inside her for 9 months until their baby is born.

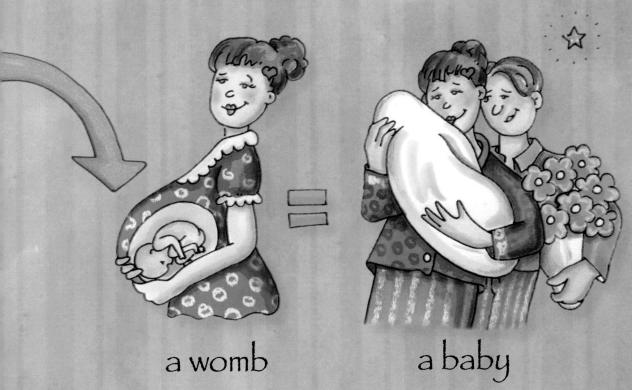

a womb   a baby

Surrogate recipe

Sometimes Mummy's womb doesn't work properly even though her eggs and Daddy's sperms are alright, so they need another woman's womb to grow their baby for them for 9 months.

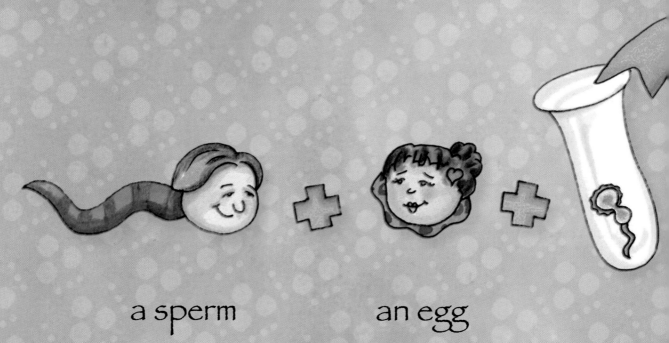

a sperm   an egg

In this case, the doctor fertilizes Mummy's egg and Daddy's sperm in a test tube and then places the embryo in another woman's womb. When it is born she gives Mummy and Daddy their baby.

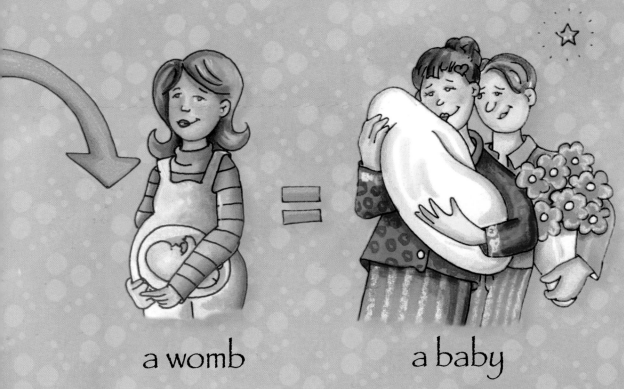

a womb   a baby

Adoption recipe

The missing ingredients in this recipe may vary, sometimes it is Daddy's sperms that don't work or sometimes it is Mummy's eggs or maybe her womb, and many times not even the doctors know what the real problem was.

Sometimes Mummy and Daddy want to adopt even if they have had children with the classical recipe before.

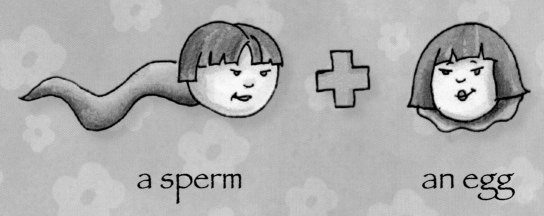

a sperm   an egg

In this recipe all the ingredients: the egg and the sperm and the womb come from another man and woman, who have the baby using the classical recipe.
The baby is given to Mummy and Daddy in adoption when it is born or sometimes when it is a little older.

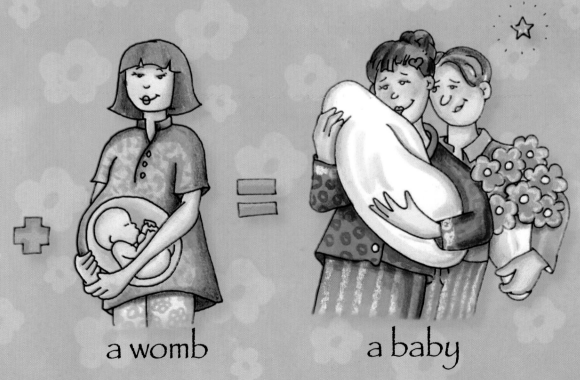

a womb   a baby

29

The families

Nowadays families are formed in many different ways. No one is better than the other, they are only different.

Sometimes families have lots and lots of children and some just have one.

Sometimes parents divorce and then remarry and suddenly you might have more brothers and sisters, sometimes they get divorced and you have none.

Sometimes parents are young and sometimes they are older.

Sometimes families only have one parent, which could be either a Mummy or a Daddy and some families are made of couples with no children at all.

Every family have their children using one of the recipes described. So your friend, your neighbour, your teacher, your parents, everyone around you was born from one of them.

No matter with which recipe you were born or how you came into Mummy and Daddy's arms, they love you just the same because they had been longing for you to be part of their family.

We are all special and unique no matter how we were made or conceived.

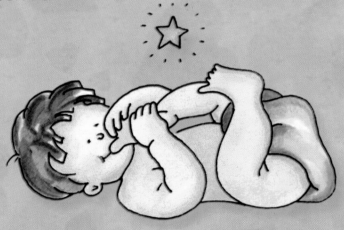

The birth of a baby in itself is a miracle ...
So we are all little miracles of life.